WEIGHT LOSS SUCCESS STORIES

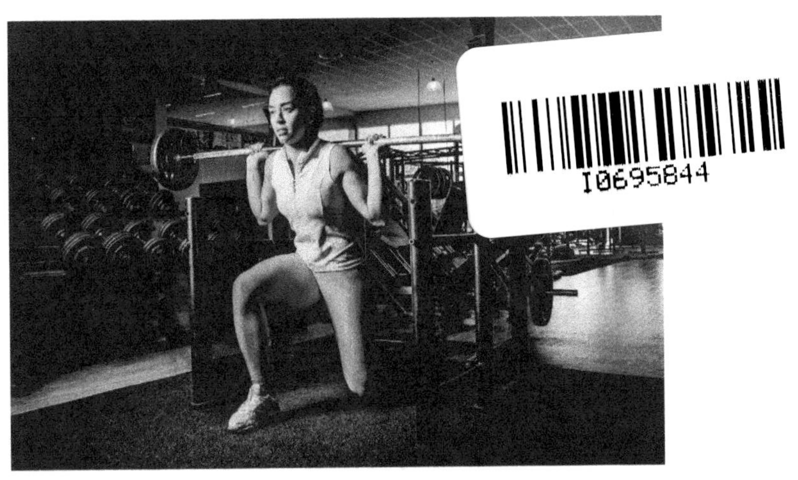

Real People's, Real Results,
The Tips And Guides For The
20st ERA

ANTHONY A. CANGELOSI

Table of Contents

INTRODUCTION

Quite a long time ago, in a little curious town named Ponderdale, carried on with a man named Oliver. Oliver had consistently battled with his weight and had attempted endless eating regimens and work-out schedules, yet none appeared to work. Baffled and crippled, he wandered the town capriciously, expecting an answer.

One radiant evening, as Oliver walked around the roads, he coincidentally found a curious little bookshop concealed in a corner. The sign hanging outside read, "The Book Niche: Where Words Change Lives." Captivated, he entered the charming store, welcomed by the smell of old books and the delicate song of traditional music playing behind the scenes.

As Oliver investigated the shelves, he saw a little segment devoted to wellbeing and health. His eyes chose a fascinating book with a title that ignited his interest: "Weight reduction Examples of overcoming adversity through Perusing." Suspicious yet captivated, he opened the book to find a prelude composed by the writer, a famous wellbeing master named Dr. Amelia Summers.

Dr. Summers made sense of how she had led broad examination on the force of the brain and its impact on weight reduction. She saw that people who submerged themselves in books' reality, stories, and encounters connected with weight reduction started to adap

Welcome To Weight reduction example of overcoming adversity, where you will take illustrations and have an extreme advisers for drove you to the achievement.

In our current reality where cheap food chains rule traffic intersections and stationary ways of life have turned into the standard, the battle to shed abundance weight has turned into a regular fight for endless people. We have all seen the force of assurance, saw somebody who has lost a huge measure of weight, and have wondered about their extraordinary change. It is inside these moving accounts of flexibility, win, and change that we track down trust and inspiration to leave on our own weight reduction venture.

This weight reduction examples of overcoming adversity book gathers an assortment of exceptional records from people who have assumed command over their lives and accomplished momentous weight reduction objectives. In every story, an individual excursion unfurls - one that uncovers the crude feelings, traps, and wins experienced en route. These accounts act as a demonstration of the unstoppable human soul and show that arriving at our weight reduction objectives isn't just imaginable yet inside our grip.

Through these pages, you will observer the hardships of conventional individuals who, outfitted with desire, devotion, and steady assurance, started their weight reduction venture. As you dive into every exceptional story, you will track down examples to execute, motivation to fuel your fire, and functional tips to help you.

HISTORY OF FIVE REAL PEOPLE'S THAT SUCCESS

1) Sarah: the Social Media Superstar: Sarah was just like any other typical Instagram user until she decided to document her weight loss journey. She started with a few followers, but as she began sharing her progress pictures, workout routines, and healthy recipes, her account exploded with thousands of followers. Sarah's captivating before-and-after pictures showcased her dedication and motivated others to follow suit. She became an inspiration to many, gaining media attention and landing endorsement deals with fitness brands. Today, she continues to influence her followers, spreading the message of self-love and perseverance.

2) Mike, the Motivated Marathon Runner: Mike was known in his small town for his love of junk food and laziness. However, when his best friend was diagnosed with a weight-related illness, it was a wake-up call for him. Determined to turn his life around, Mike started running. He began with a simple goal of running a mile without stopping but soon discovered a passion for long-distance running. Mike's journey to fitness was closely followed by his local newspaper, and soon his story spread like wildfire. He completed multiple marathons, inspiring others to lace up their shoes and start running for their health. His remarkable transformation earned him the nickname "The Marathon Marvel."

3) Emily, the Celebrity Chef: Emily was a well-known chef with a television show focused on indulgent recipes and comfort food. However, she decided she wanted to set an example for her viewers by adopting a healthier lifestyle. Emily started experimenting with healthy alternatives to her decadent dishes and showcased them on her show. Her audience was captivated and couldn't wait to try out her easy-to-follow recipes. Emily's weight loss transformation was heavily covered by media outlets, and she became a leading figure in the movement towards nutritious yet delicious cooking. Her cooking show evolved and became an influential platform for promoting health-conscious eating.

4) Mark, the Music Maestro: Mark was a musician who struggled with his weight throughout his early career. On the brink of giving up, he decided to embark on a life-changing weight loss journey. Alongside his musical talents, Mark discovered a passion for dancing, which became an integral part of his fitness routine. Through dance, he shed the excess weight, revealing a fitter and more confident version of himself. Mark's incredible transformation caught the attention of talk shows, magazines, and even music videos. He became the symbol of embracing one's passion and transforming not only physically but also artistically. Today, Mark is renowned as the "Rhythm Rebel" both for his music and his inspiring weight loss journey.

5) Jessica, the Fashion Phenomenon: Jessica had always loved fashion but felt limited by her weight. Determined to break the stereotype that fashion was exclusively for the slim, she embarked on a weight loss journey. As the pounds dropped, Jessica's fashion sense flourished. She started a blog documenting her style evolution and promoting body positivity. Jessica caught the attention of fashion designers, who were eager to collaborate with her. Her remarkable transformation was covered by fashion magazines, showcasing her incredible sense of style and inspiring many others to embrace fashion, regardless of their size. Jessica became a fashion phenomenon, breaking barriers and elevating the message of body inclusivity within the industry.

Chapter 1: The Beginning

The start of weight reduction examples of overcoming adversity is many times set apart by a choice to roll out an improvement and assume command over one's wellbeing. An excursion requires devotion, assurance, and steadiness. This extensive substance will frame the critical stages and procedures that can assist people with beginning their weight reduction venture doing great.

1. **Put forth practical objectives:** The initial step to making weight reduction progress is laying out reasonable

objectives. It's essential to have an unmistakable comprehension of what you need to accomplish and to separate it into sensible achievements. Remember that sound weight reduction is slow, with an objective of 1-2 pounds each week.

2. Talk with a medical care proficient: Prior to beginning any get-healthy plan, it's fundamental to talk with a medical services proficient, like a specialist or an enlisted dietitian. They can give direction customized to your particular requirements, assess any basic medical issue, and guarantee that you approach weight reduction in a protected and economical way.

3. Make a decent dinner plan: A reasonable and nutritious feast plan is vital for weight reduction achievement. Center around consolidating entire food varieties, like organic products, vegetables, lean proteins, entire grains, and sound fats. Consider segment control and hold back nothing shortfall by consuming less calories than you consume.

4. Hydration: Staying hydrated is frequently neglected yet assumes a huge part in weight reduction achievement. Drinking a satisfactory measure of water can assist with supporting digestion, check hunger, and advance in general wellbeing. Go for the gold 8 glasses (64 ounces) of water each day, or more in the event that you are truly dynamic.

5. Actual work: Taking part in standard actual work is fundamental for weight reduction and in general prosperity. Go for the gold of cardiovascular activities, like strolling, running, cycling, or swimming, and strength preparing activities to assemble fit bulk. Begin with reasonable measures of activity and slowly increment power and term.

6. Find a work-out routine you appreciate: To guarantee long haul adherence to a work-out daily practice, it is essential to find proactive tasks you appreciate. Attempt various kinds of activity, for example, bunch wellness classes, sports, or outside exercises, until you find something that you anticipate doing. Different activities can assist with forestalling weariness and keep you spurred.

7. Look for help and responsibility: Encircling yourself with a strong organization can assist you with remaining propelled and responsible all through your weight reduction venture. Consider joining a weight reduction support bunch, finding a responsibility accomplice, or looking for proficient assistance from a dietitian or a fitness coach.

8. Track progress: Observing your advancement can give inspiration and assist you with remaining focused. Keep a diary or utilize a portable application to follow your food consumption, work-out schedules, and estimations. Seeing your improvement over the long run can help your certainty and drive you to keep going with solid decisions.

9. Practice careful eating: Careful eating includes focusing on the impressions of eating, like the taste, surface, and smell of food. Dial back, relish each chomp, and pay attention to your body's craving and completion prompts. This can assist forestall gorging and advance a sound connection with food.

10. Get sufficient rest: Satisfactory rest is fundamental for weight reduction achievement. Absence of rest can disturb hormonal equilibrium, increment desires for unfortunate food sources, and upset weight reduction endeavors. Hold back nothing long periods of value rest consistently to help your weight reduction objectives.

11. Remain positive and persuaded: Weight reduction excursion can have its promising and less promising times. It's essential to keep a positive outlook and remain roused in the interim. Celebrate little triumphs, practice self-empathy, and spotlight on the positive changes you are making for your wellbeing.

12. Adjust and change: Recollect that weight reduction is a customized excursion, and what works for one individual may not work for another. Be available to adjusting and changing your methodology on a case by case basis. On the off chance that a specific procedure or plan isn't yielding the ideal outcomes, don't hesitate for even a moment to take a stab at a novel, new thing. Persistent learning and trial and error are vital to finding what turns out best for your body and way of life.

13. Deal with your psychological and profound prosperity: Weight reduction isn't just about actual changes; it likewise includes dealing with your psychological and close to home prosperity. Practice pressure the board strategies, like contemplation, yoga, or journaling. Look for help from a specialist or guide if necessary, as profound eating or hidden mental variables can influence weight reduction endeavors.

14. Celebrate non-scale triumphs: Recollect that weight reduction achievement still up in the air by the number on the scale. Celebrate non-scale triumphs, for example, expanded energy levels, further developed mind-set, better rest, or arriving at wellness achievements. These accomplishments are similarly significant and act major areas of strength for as to continue onward.

15. Keep a drawn out viewpoint: Finally, it's essential to take on a drawn out point of view on your weight reduction venture. Practical weight reduction isn't about convenient solutions or fleeting eating regimens. It's tied in with making enduring way of life changes that advance by and large wellbeing and prosperity. Embrace the excursion, show restraint toward yourself, and spotlight on embracing a better way of life instead of simply accomplishing a particular number on the scale.

the start of weight reduction examples of overcoming adversity begins with a choice to roll out an improvement, combined with practical objectives, a decent feast plan, ordinary actual work, support, following advancement, and a positive mentality. Make sure to zero in on by and large wellbeing and prosperity, celebrate non-scale triumphs, and keep a drawn out viewpoint. By following these techniques and remaining committed, you are getting yourself positioned for an effective weight reduction venture.

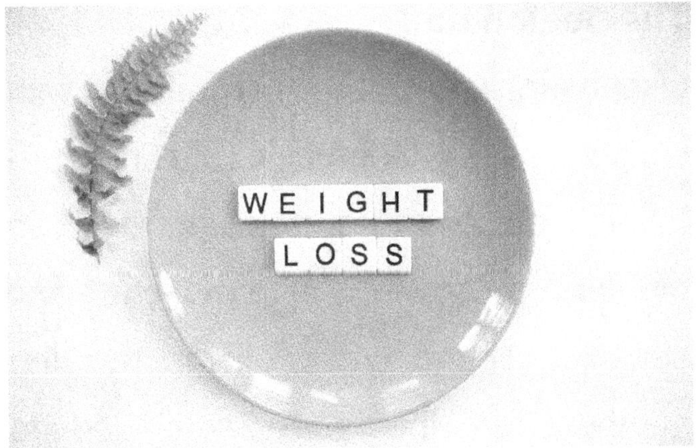

My Struggle with Weight

Weight, it is a constant companion that has followed me throughout my life. From an early age, I found myself battling with the scales, facing the never-ending cycle of losing and gaining weight. However, through persistence, determination, and a shift in mindset, I managed to transform my struggle into a weight loss success story, brimming with hope and inspiration.

The Beginning:

Like countless others, my journey with weight issues began in childhood. I found solace in food, using it as a means to cope with emotions and stress. As the years went by, the numbers on the scale continued to climb, and with them came a myriad of health complications and diminished self-confidence.

Acknowledging the Problem:

It took a significant moment of realization for me to acknowledge that my relationship with food was unhealthy and that I needed to make a change. I asked myself the hard questions and confronted the deeper reasons behind my struggle with weight. This introspection laid the foundation for my transformation.

Road to change:Weight loss success stories often begin with a road to change. This road is different for each individual, but some common themes emerge as people embark on their journey to reach their goal weight and maintain a healthier lifestyle.

Road To Change:

One important aspect of this road to change is making the decision to start. This decision can be spurred by a variety of factors, such as wanting to improve overall health, boost self-confidence, or increase energy levels. Once the decision is made, individuals often have to mentally prepare themselves for the challenges that lie ahead.

Another crucial step is setting realistic and achievable goals. It is important to recognize that losing weight takes time and effort, and it is unlikely that results will be seen overnight. By setting smaller, attainable goals along the way, individuals can experience success and stay motivated to continue their journey.

Implementing a healthy eating plan is also a fundamental part of the road to change. This may involve learning how to make nutritious food choices, portion control, and cooking meals at home to have more control over ingredients and preparation methods. It may also involve seeking support from registered dietitians or nutritionists to develop a personalized meal plan.

Regular physical activity is another essential component of the road to change. Finding activities that are enjoyable and sustainable is key to sticking with an exercise routine. This may involve trying out different types of exercise, such as walking, running, weightlifting, swimming, or yoga, to find what works best for the individual.

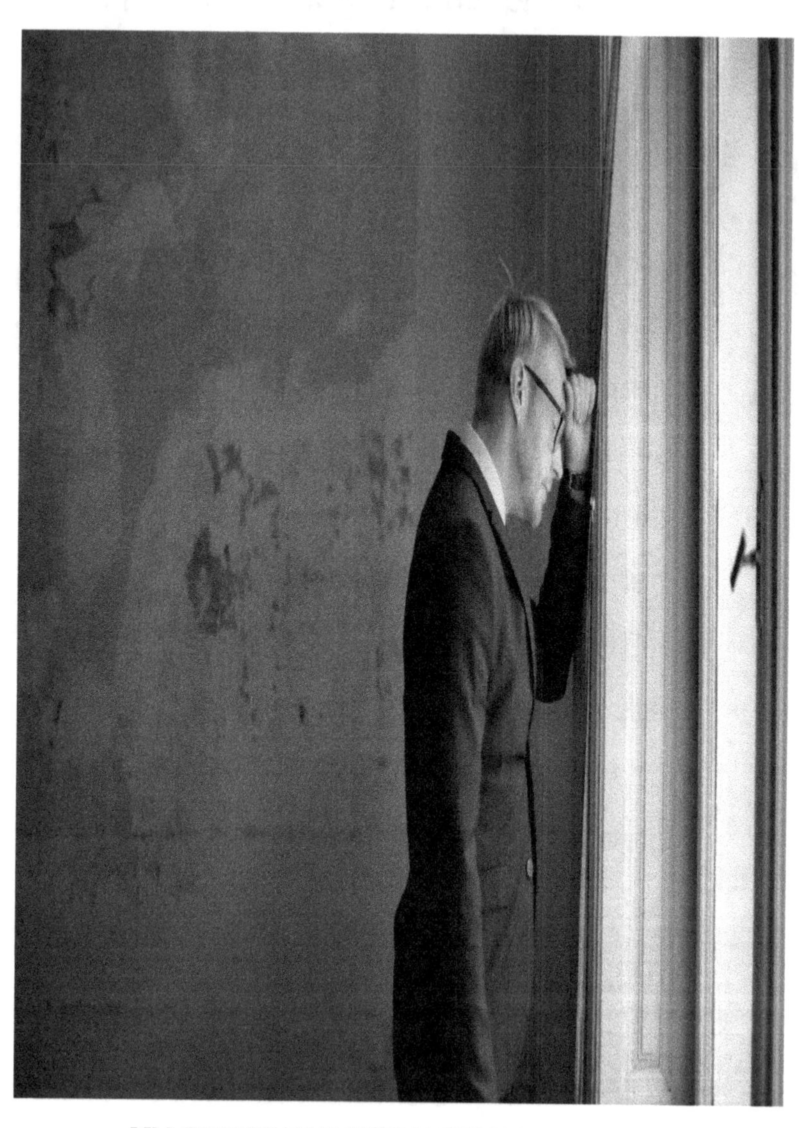

MY STRUGGLE WITH WEIGHT

Chapter 2: Realization

Realization serves as a powerful catalyst for change. It is the moment when individuals truly comprehend the negative consequences and implications of their unhealthy choices. Different individuals experience this realization in varying ways, but the impact is undeniable. Realization often drives a deep internal shift in mentality, leading to the development of determination, motivation, and accountability—an essential foundation for long-term weight loss success.

Types of Realizations in Weight Loss Success Stories:

1. Impact on Health:

Many weight loss success stories feature individuals who undergo a decisive moment of realization connected to their health. Symptoms such as high blood pressure, diabetes, chronic fatigue, or physical pain are often the awakening triggers. Through personal testimony or medical diagnosis, people are forced to confront the real disparities between their current lifestyle and the health they desire. Realizing the severe health risks associated with obesity resonates deeply and becomes a catalyst for change.

2. Physical Limitations and Mobility Issues:

For some individuals, the realization occurs when their weight starts inhibiting their ability to engage in activities they used to enjoy. This realization, often accompanied by the experience of being unable to perform even simple physical tasks with ease, helps individuals see the direct impact of excess weight on their quality of life. This can motivate them to make changes to regain mobility, independence, and the freedom to participate fully in daily activities.

3. Mental and Emotional Well-being:

Apart from physical health, weight loss success stories also frequently involve mental and emotional realization. Many individuals come to a point of recognizing that their weight is linked to feelings of low self-esteem, lack of confidence, and even depression. This realization sparks a desire to improve their overall well-being and regain self-worth. Acknowledging the significant impact of their weight on their emotions fosters a mental mindset necessary for healthy weight loss success.

4. External Influences and Social Interactions:

Sometimes, realization is prompted by external factors. These can include comments from friends, family, or loved ones regarding weight or appearance. Cruel remarks or insensitive jokes can be painful in the moment, but serve as a reality check that motivates change. The desire to feel accepted, confident in social settings, or be a role model for loved ones can also initiate the realization prompting individuals to begin their weight loss journey.

Realization is an essential aspect of weight loss success stories as it ignites within individuals the motivation and drive needed to make sustainable and meaningful change. While different factors contribute to personal awakenings, the critical element is a deep understanding of the consequences of unhealthy behaviors and decisions. Whether the realization stems from health concerns, physical limitations, mental well-being, or social influences, it serves as a turning point that propels individuals towards positive transformation. Recognition of these significant realizations underscores the power and impact of determination, a sound plan, a support system, and perseverance that drives long-lasting weight loss success.

The Turning Point

Weight reduction can be a difficult excursion for some people. It requires devotion, discipline, and persistence to accomplish economical outcomes. Notwithstanding, there frequently comes a defining moment in weight reduction examples of overcoming adversity that fills in as an impetus for people to roll out significant improvements in their way of life and at last accomplish their objectives. In this article, we will investigate the different parts of this defining moment, from the encounters that trigger it to the moves made to guarantee long haul achievement.

1. Acknowledgment of the issue:

The defining moment in a weight reduction example of overcoming adversity frequently starts with the individual perceiving that they have a weight issue and recognizing the adverse consequence it has on their general wellbeing and prosperity. This acknowledgment could come from various elements - feeling awkward in their own skin, getting a reminder from a medical services proficient, or encountering torment and distress because of overabundance weight.

2. Inspiration and objective setting:

When the issue is recognized, people track down the inspiration to begin their weight reduction venture. It could be started by a huge occasion, like a wedding or a gathering, or basically the craving to carry on with a better, seriously satisfying life. Putting forth practical objectives is likewise essential in this stage, as it assists people with characterizing what they need to accomplish and keeps them engaged and responsible in the meantime.

3. Seeking Support and direction:

A pivotal component in the defining moment of weight reduction examples of overcoming adversity is looking for help and direction from experts or emotionally supportive networks. This might include talking with an enrolled dietitian or nutritionist to make a customized feast plan, joining a weight reduction support gathering, or in any event, employing a fitness coach.

Having somebody to guide and support them all through their process can altogether build the odds of coming out on top.

4. Embracing better dietary patterns:

One more significant part of the defining moment in weight reduction examples of overcoming adversity is the reception of better dietary patterns. This normally includes a shift towards an even and supplement thick eating routine that incorporates natural products, vegetables, lean proteins, entire grains, and sound fats. Segment control and careful eating are likewise underscored to foster a better relationship with food and diminish the propensity to gorge or enjoy undesirable decisions.

5. Consolidating normal actual work:

Active work assumes a crucial part in weight reduction examples of overcoming adversity. The defining moment frequently includes integrating ordinary activity into one's day to day daily schedule. Whether it's strolling, running, cycling, or participating in wellness classes, customary active work assists consume calories, work with muscling, and further develop by and large wellness levels. Finding an action that one appreciates makes it simpler to adhere to a steady work-out everyday practice.

6. Defeating snags and mishaps:

Weight reduction ventures are seldom going great, and people might experience hindrances and misfortunes en route. The defining moment in examples of overcoming adversity includes gaining from misfortunes and tracking down the inspiration to conquer them. It's significant to see mishaps as learning open doors instead of disappointments and to foster versatility and assurance to keep pursuing a definitive objective.

7. Embracing a manageable way of life:

Maybe the main defining moment in weight reduction examples of overcoming adversity is the change from considering weight reduction to be a transient objective to embracing a feasible and sound way of life. This includes creating solid propensities like careful eating, normal activity, and keeping a positive mentality about long haul changes. It's essential to comprehend that weight reduction is definitely not a one-time accomplishment yet a continuous interaction that requires consistency and commitment.

the defining moment in weight reduction examples of overcoming adversity is a vital second where people perceive their weight issue, track down the inspiration to change, look for help and direction, take on better propensities, defeat difficulties, and eventually embrace a feasible way of life. By making these strides, people can accomplish their weight reduction objectives and keep up with their advancement over the long haul.

Chapter 3: Setting Goals

Setting weight loss goals and achieving them has been a common struggle for many people over the years. However, past individuals who have successfully met their weight loss goals can provide inspiration and insight into effective strategies and equipment that can make the process easier. In this article, we will discuss a few of the most well-known success stories and the equipment they used to facilitate their weight loss journey.

1. Oprah Winfrey:

Oprah Winfrey, a media mogul, has openly discussed her struggles with weight loss throughout her life. However, in recent years, she has made significant progress in maintaining a healthier weight. One of the easiest equipment she attributes to her success is a wearable fitness tracker. These devices, such as Fitbit or Apple Watch, help individuals track their daily steps, calories burned, and heart rate. Monitoring these metrics can provide a tangible way to measure progress and motivate oneself to stay active.

2. Jared Fogle:

Jared Fogle, the former spokesperson for Subway, became an icon in the weight loss industry for losing a substantial amount of weight by eating Subway sandwiches. While his story is controversial due to subsequent legal issues, his initial weight loss journey is worth mentioning. Fogle often emphasized the importance of portion control and made use of a simple kitchen scale. Using a kitchen scale allows individuals to accurately measure food portions and ensure they are consuming the right amount of calories. This can be especially helpful for individuals who tend to overeat or struggle with estimating portion sizes.

3. Chris Powell:

Chris Powell, a personal trainer and host of the TV show "Extreme Weight Loss," has helped numerous individuals achieve their weight loss goals. One piece of equipment he frequently highlights is resistance bands. Resistance bands are a versatile and affordable tool that can be used for strength training exercises targeting various muscle groups. They are portable and easy to use, making them ideal for individuals looking to incorporate strength training into their weight loss routine without investing in heavy gym equipment.

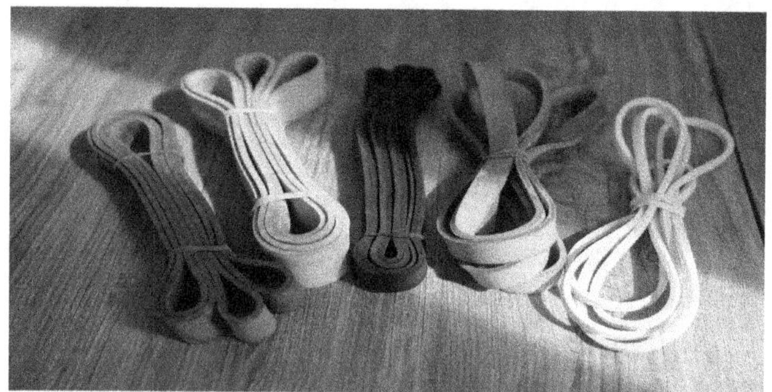

4. Richard Simmons:

Richard Simmons, a well-known fitness guru and motivational speaker, has been inspiring people to lose weight for decades. While his approach might be seen as unconventional, his success lies in the simplicity of his exercise equipment of choice: a basic step platform. Step platforms are widely available and allow individuals to perform various cardiovascular exercises and aerobic routines. They provide an efficient way to burn calories and improve cardiovascular fitness levels right in the comfort of one's own home.

5. Marie Osmond:

Marie Osmond, a singer and actress, has struggled with weight fluctuations throughout her career. However, she successfully lost weight and maintained it with the help of a home treadmill. Treadmills offer a convenient way to incorporate cardio exercise into a weight loss routine. They are versatile, allowing individuals to walk, jog, or run at their own pace, and often come equipped with features like incline settings and pre-programmed workouts, providing a challenging yet customizable fitness experience.

past individuals who have achieved success in weight loss have utilized a range of equipment to support their journey. From wearable fitness trackers to kitchen scales, resistance bands, step platforms, and treadmills, each equipment serves a purpose in facilitating weight loss and making the process easier. However, it is important to note that while equipment can be helpful, consistent effort, a balanced diet, and a commitment to overall lifestyle changes are essential for long-term success in weight loss.

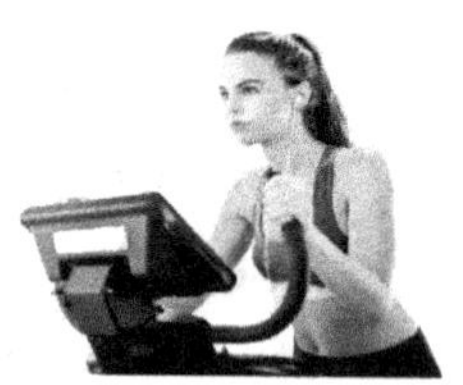

Treadmills

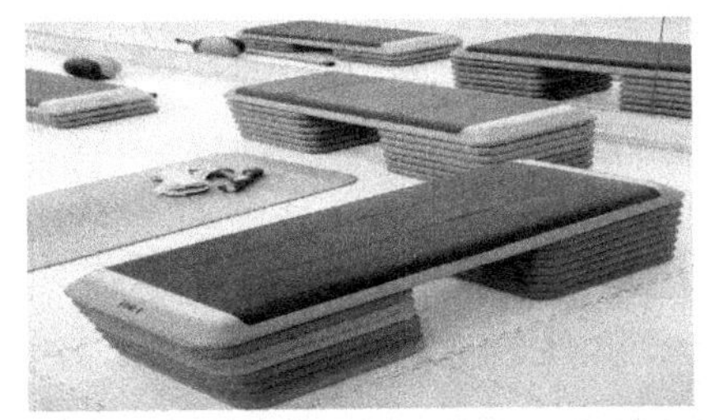

Step platform

Creating a Vision for Success

Creating a vision for success on weight loss involves setting clear and specific goals, developing a positive mindset, and implementing effective strategies to achieve those goals. This comprehensive guide will provide you with the necessary steps and strategies to create a vision for success on your weight loss journey.

1. Define Your "Why":

To create a powerful vision for weight loss success, it's essential to understand your reasons for embarking on this journey. Take time to reflect on why losing weight is important to you. Is it for health reasons, to boost your self-confidence, or to improve your overall quality of life? Clearly identifying your "why" will serve as the foundation for your vision and provide motivation when facing challenges.

2.Define Your Goals:

The second thing in creating a vision for success on weight loss is to define your goals. Set clear and specific goals that align with your desired weight, fitness level, and overall health. For example, you might set a goal to lose 20 pounds in the next three months or to fit into a specific dress size.

3. Visualize Your Success:

Once you have defined your goals, it's important to visualize your success. Take a moment to imagine yourself achieving your goals and how it will feel once you have reached your ideal weight. Visualizing success helps to create a positive mindset and keeps you motivated throughout your weight loss journey.

4. Develop a Positive Mindset:
Creating a positive mindset is crucial for long-term success in weight loss. Instead of focusing on the obstacles or setbacks you may encounter, focus on the progress you have made and the positive changes you are experiencing. Adopting a positive mindset helps to overcome self-doubt, stay motivated, and persevere in the face of challenges.

5. Set Realistic and Measurable Milestones:
To create a vision for success in weight loss, it's important to set realistic and measurable milestones. Break down your ultimate goal into smaller,

achievable milestones, such as losing a certain number of pounds each month or increasing your workout duration gradually. These milestones will keep you motivated as you achieve them, and also help you track your progress.

6. Create a Plan:

Having a well-structured plan is crucial for success in weight loss. Develop a meal plan that includes nutritious and balanced meals, and set aside time for regular physical activity. Consider consulting with a nutritionist or a fitness expert to help create a personalized plan that caters to your specific needs and goals.

7. Implement Healthy Habits:

Creating a vision for success on weight loss involves implementing healthy habits that support your goals. This includes making healthy food choices, staying hydrated, getting enough sleep, and maintaining a consistent exercise routine. These habits not only support weight loss but also promote overall well-being.

8. Monitor Your Progress:

Regularly monitor your progress to stay accountable and motivated. Use tools such as a food diary, a fitness tracker, or a weekly weigh-in to track your progress and identify areas that need improvement. Celebrate your achievements along the way to stay motivated and reinforce positive behaviors.

9. Seek Support:

Having a support system can greatly enhance your chances of success in weight loss. Seek support from family, friends, or join a support group to share your challenges and victories. Consider partnering with a weight loss coach or a personal trainer who can provide guidance, motivation, and accountability.

10. Stay Resilient:

Creating a vision for success on weight loss requires resilience. There may be times when you face setbacks or challenges, but it's important to stay focused, learn from any mistakes, and keep moving forward. Remind yourself of your ultimate vision and why achieving it is important to you.

11. Celebrate Your Achievements:

Lastly, celebrate your achievements along the way. Recognize your hard work, dedication, and the progress you have made. Reward yourself with non-food-related treats, such as a spa day, a new outfit, or a weekend getaway. Celebrating your achievements reinforces positive behaviors and motivates you to continue working towards your ultimate vision.

creating a vision for success on weight loss involves setting clear goals, visualizing success, developing a positive mindset, and implementing effective strategies. By following these steps and staying committed to your vision, you can achieve long-term tosuccess in your weight loss journey.

Chapter 4: Knowledge is Power

When it comes to weight loss, knowledge is indeed power. It is essential to understand the science behind weight loss and how various factors contribute to our overall health and body composition. Armed with this knowledge, individuals can make informed decisions and implement effective strategies to achieve their weight loss goals. In this article, we will explore why knowledge is power in weight loss and how it can help you on your journey to a healthier and slimmer body.

Understanding the Science: Weight loss is not simply about cutting calories or exercising more. It is a complex process that involves the interplay of various factors, such as metabolism, hormonal balance, and genetics. By educating yourself about how these factors affect weight loss, you can develop a more comprehensive and targeted approach to your journey. For example, knowing that certain foods can boost your metabolism or that resistance training helps build lean muscle mass can guide your dietary choices and exercise routine.

Setting Realistic Goals: Many people embark on weight loss journeys with unrealistic expectations. They might aim to lose an excessive amount of weight within a short period, only to get discouraged and give up when they don't see immediate results. Knowledge about healthy and sustainable weight loss can help you set realistic goals and avoid falling into the trap of crash diets or extreme workouts. Understanding that slow and steady progress is more likely to lead to long-term success can keep you motivated and focused on your goals.

Making Informed Dietary Choices: The abundance of information available about nutrition can be overwhelming, but having basic knowledge about macronutrients, vitamins, and minerals is crucial for weight loss. Understanding how different nutrients impact your body can help you make informed choices about the foods you consume. For example, knowing that protein is essential for muscle growth and repair can help you prioritize protein-rich foods and regulate your appetite. Additionally, having knowledge about portion sizes and calorie content can enable you to make sensible decisions when dining out or grocery shopping.

Implementing Effective Exercise Routines: Exercise plays a vital role in weight loss, but not all exercises are equally effective. Educating yourself about different types of workouts, such as cardio, strength training, and high-intensity interval training (HIIT), can help you design a well-rounded exercise routine that maximizes calorie burn and builds lean muscle mass. Understanding the concept of progressive overload and how it contributes to muscle growth can ensure that you consistently challenge your body and avoid hitting plateaus in your fitness progress.

Developing Healthy Habits: Knowledge about weight loss goes beyond just the physical aspects. It also involves cultivating healthy habits and behaviors that support long-term success. Understanding the psychological and emotional factors that contribute to weight gain and overeating can help you address any underlying issues and develop strategies to overcome them. Knowledge about stress management, mindful eating, and healthy sleep patterns can also play a significant role in weight loss.

Staying Motivated and Accountable:
Finally, knowledge is power when it comes to staying motivated and accountable on your weight loss journey. By continuously learning about the latest research and evidence-based practices, you can stay up to date with new strategies and techniques. Moreover, educating yourself about the success stories of others who have achieved their weight loss goals can serve as inspiration and keep you motivated during challenging times.

knowledge is power in weight loss. Understanding the science behind weight loss, setting realistic goals, making informed dietary choices, implementing effective exercise routines, developing healthy habits, and staying motivated and accountable are all crucial aspects of successful weight loss. By continually seeking knowledge and applying it to your journey, you can take control of your weight, enhance your overall wellness, and achieve long-term success in reaching your desired body composition. Remember, the power to transform lies within your hands, and knowledge is the key that unlocks it.

Understanding the Science of Weight Loss

Weight loss is a common goal for many people, but understanding the science behind it can be crucial for achieving long-lasting results. The process of shedding excess weight involves a complex interplay of various factors, including diet, exercise, metabolism, and genetics. By exploring the science behind weight loss, individuals can gain a deeper understanding of the mechanisms at play and make more informed decisions about their journey towards a healthier body.

1. Energy Balance:

The fundamental principle behind weight loss is the concept of energy balance. It refers to the relationship between the energy consumed through food and the energy expended by the body. If the calories consumed exceed the calories burned, the excess energy is stored as fat, resulting in weight gain. Conversely, if the calories burned exceed the calories consumed, the body taps into its fat stores to make up for the energy deficit, leading to weight loss.

2. Caloric Deficit:

To create a caloric deficit and promote weight loss, individuals typically need to consume fewer calories than their body requires. This can be achieved through a combination of reduced calorie intake and increased physical activity. It is important to note that creating a healthy caloric deficit is essential as severe calorie restriction can lead to nutrient deficiencies and metabolic slowdown.

3. Diet:

The type and quality of the food we consume play a crucial role in weight loss. A well-balanced diet should focus on nutrient-dense foods such as fruits, vegetables, lean proteins, whole grains, and healthy fats. These foods provide essential vitamins, minerals, and fiber while keeping the individual satiated. Additionally, reducing intake of high-calorie, processed foods and sugary beverages can aid in creating a caloric deficit.

4. Exercise:

Regular physical activity is crucial for weight loss as it helps increase caloric expenditure, build lean muscle mass, and improve overall health. Both aerobic exercise, such as running or swimming, and strength training, such as weightlifting or resistance exercises, have their own unique benefits. Aerobic exercise burns calories, improves cardiovascular health, and boosts metabolism, while strength training builds muscle, increases metabolism, and improves body composition.

5. Metabolism:

One important factor affecting weight loss is metabolism, which refers to the complex biochemical processes in the body that convert food into energy. Many factors influence metabolism, including age, sex, genetics, body composition, and hormone levels. While it is true that some individuals may have a naturally faster or slower metabolism, the impact of metabolism on weight loss is often overstated. In reality, it is the overall energy balance that determines weight loss or gain.

6. Genetics:

Genetics can influence an individual's predisposition to gaining or losing weight. Some people may have a genetic tendency to store more fat or have a slower metabolism. However, while genetics may play a role, they do not dictate a person's weight destiny. With the right lifestyle changes, including a healthy diet and regular exercise, individuals can override their genetic predispositions and achieve weight loss.

7. Sustainable Weight Loss:

The key to successful weight loss lies in adopting sustainable lifestyle changes rather than resorting to crash diets or quick fixes. A gradual and steady weight loss of 1-2 pounds per week is considered healthy and more likely to be maintained long-term. It is also important to emphasize behavior change and develop healthy habits, such as mindful eating, portion control, and regular physical activity, which can be sustained over a lifetime.

understanding the science behind weight loss can empower individuals to make informed decisions about their diet, exercise routine, and overall lifestyle. By focusing on creating a caloric deficit through a balanced diet and regular exercise, individuals can achieve sustainable weight loss and improve their overall health and well-being. Remember, weight loss is a journey that requires patience, perseverance, and a commitment to making lasting changes.

Chapter5:Overcoming Obstacles

Losing weight is a common goal for many people, but it can also be a challenging journey filled with obstacles. Whether it's a lack of motivation, social pressures, or unrealistic expectations, there are many roadblocks that can hinder your progress. However, with the right mindset and strategies, you can overcome these obstacles and achieve your weight loss goals. In this comprehensive guide, we will explore some of the most common obstacles in weight loss and provide practical tips on how to overcome them.

1. Lack of Motivation: One of the biggest obstacles in weight loss is a lack of motivation. When the initial excitement wears off, it can be difficult to stay focused and committed to your goals. To overcome this obstacle, it's important to find your "why" - the reason why you want to lose weight and improve your health. Whether it's to feel more confident, improve your overall well-being, or set a positive example for your loved ones, identifying your motivation can provide you with the drive to keep going. Additionally, setting short-term goals and celebrating small victories along the way can help boost your motivation.

2. Unrealistic Expectations: Another common obstacle in weight loss is setting unrealistic expectations. Many people have a tendency to expect immediate results, which can lead to disappointment and frustration. It's essential to understand that weight loss is a gradual process and that sustainable results take time. Setting realistic and achievable goals, such as losing 1-2 pounds per week, can help you stay focused and maintain a positive mindset. Remember, slow and steady progress is more likely to lead to long-term success.

3. Social Pressures: Social pressures can be a significant obstacle in weight loss, especially when it comes to social gatherings, dining out, and peer influence. It's important to communicate your goals and boundaries with your friends and family. Let them know why your health is important to you and ask for their support. If you're attending a social event, consider bringing a healthy dish to share or eating a small, nutritious meal beforehand to avoid overindulging. Surrounding yourself with like-minded individuals or finding an accountability partner can also help you stay on track despite social pressures.

4. Emotional Eating: Emotional eating is a common obstacle that many people face during their weight loss journey. Stress, boredom, sadness, and other emotions can trigger overeating or indulging in unhealthy foods. Developing healthy coping mechanisms, such as practicing mindfulness, engaging in physical activity, or seeking support from a therapist or support group, can help you overcome emotional eating. It's also essential to create a healthy relationship with food by focusing on nourishing your body rather than using it as a source of comfort or stress relief.

5. Plateaus: Plateaus, where weight loss stalls even with continued efforts, can be demotivating and challenging to overcome. To break through a plateau, consider making adjustments to your diet and exercise routine. This could include increasing your physical activity, experimenting with different workouts, or modifying your calorie intake. Additionally, keeping track of your food intake and monitoring portion sizes can help identify any areas where you may be consuming more calories than you realize. Remember that plateaus are normal and part of the weight loss process, so don't get discouraged. Stay patient and trust the process.

6. Lack of Time: Many individuals struggle with finding the time to prioritize their health and weight loss goals due to busy schedules and other commitments. However, it's essential to make self-care a priority and carve out time for physical activity and meal preparation. Look for opportunities to incorporate exercise into your daily routine, such as taking the stairs instead of the elevator or going for a walk during your lunch break. Planning meals in advance and opting for quick and healthy options can also save time in the kitchen. Remember, even small pockets of time dedicated to your well-being can make a significant impact in the long run.

overcoming obstacles in weight loss requires a combination of mindset shifts, practical strategies, and consistent effort. By identifying your motivation, setting realistic goals, seeking support, and making necessary adjustments along the way, you can overcome any obstacles that come your way. Remember to celebrate your progress and focus on the positive changes you are making, both physically and mentally. With determination and perseverance, you can achieve your weight loss goals and improve your overall well-being.

Dealing with Emotional and Physical Challenges

Losing weight can be a challenging journey, both emotionally and physically. It is important to be prepared and equipped with the right strategies to overcome these challenges and achieve weight loss success. Here are some tips and techniques for dealing with emotional and physical challenges in your weight loss journey:

Emotional Challenges:

1. Set Realistic Goals: One of the biggest emotional challenges people face during weight loss is setting unrealistic goals. It is essential to set achievable and realistic goals to avoid disappointment and frustration. Break down your weight loss goals into smaller, manageable targets.

2. Stay Positive: Surround yourself with positivity and motivational resources. Read success stories of others who have achieved weight loss, follow inspirational social media accounts, and remind yourself of the reasons why you want to lose weight.

3. Practice Self-Love: Learn to love and appreciate yourself throughout your weight loss journey. Don't focus solely on the numbers on the scale, but also celebrate non-scale victories such as improved energy levels, increased stamina, and feeling more confident in your body.

4. Manage Stress: Emotional eating is a common response to stress. Find healthy ways to manage stress, such as exercise, meditation, deep breathing, or engaging in hobbies that bring you joy. Avoid using food as a source of comfort.

5. Seek Support: Surround yourself with a support system of friends, family, or even a weight loss support group. Having someone to talk to about your struggles, successes, and challenges can provide you with much-needed encouragement and motivation.

Physical Challenges:

1. Create a Balanced Diet: Focus on creating a balanced diet that includes a variety of nutrient-dense foods such as fruits, vegetables, whole grains, lean proteins, and healthy fats. Avoid crash diets or extreme calorie restrictions, as they can lead to nutrient deficiencies and have negative impacts on your overall health.

2. Find an Exercise Routine that Fits Your Lifestyle: Incorporate regular physical activity into your routine. Find activities that you enjoy, whether it's walking, dancing, swimming, or weightlifting. Experiment with different forms of exercise until you find something that you genuinely enjoy and can stick to in the long term.

3. Stay Consistent: Consistency is key when it comes to weight loss. Stay committed to your diet and exercise routine, even on days when you lack motivation or face challenges. Consistency will help you build discipline and ultimately achieve your goals.

4. Stay Hydrated: Drinking enough water is crucial for weight loss success. Water helps boost metabolism, suppress appetite, and flush out toxins from the body. Aim to drink at least eight glasses of water per day.

5. Track Your Progress: Keep track of your progress to stay motivated and accountable. Use a journal or a weight loss app to record your food intake, exercise routines, and measurements. Tracking your progress can help you identify patterns, make necessary adjustments, and celebrate milestones along the way.

Dealing with emotional and physical challenges on your weight loss journey can be tough, but with the right mindset, strategies, and support, you can overcome them and achieve weight loss success. Remember to be patient and kind to yourself, and celebrate every step of progress you make.

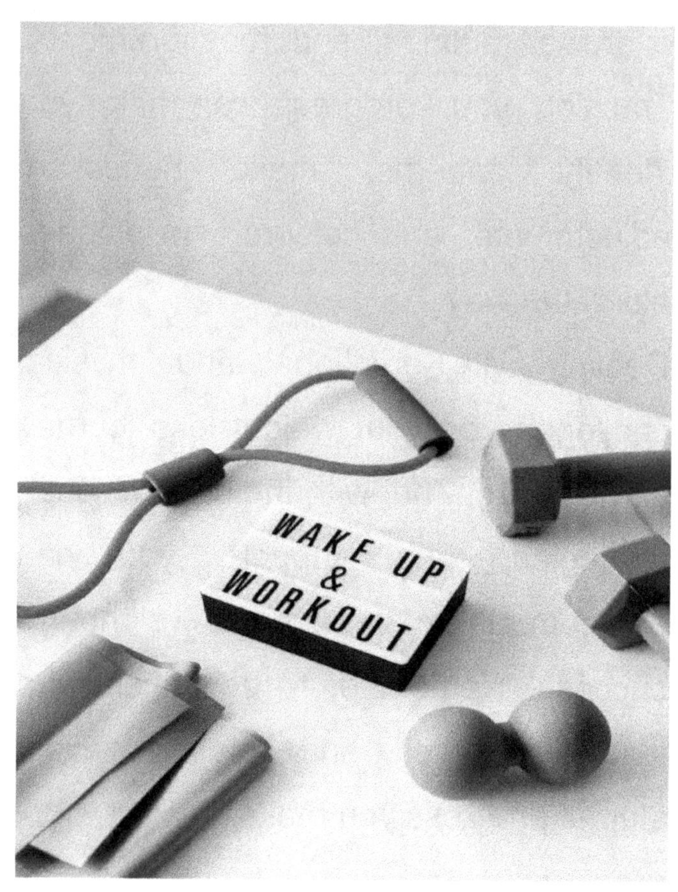

WAKE UP
&
WORKOUT

CHAPTER 6: THE POWER OF NUTRITION

Nutrition plays a crucial role in weight loss. In fact, it is often said that weight loss is 80% nutrition and 20% exercise. While exercise is important for overall health and fitness, it is the choices we make in the kitchen that truly make the difference when it comes to shedding pounds.

Eating a balanced and nutrient-rich diet not only helps in weight loss but also improves overall health and wellbeing. Here are some key reasons why nutrition is so powerful in the journey towards weight loss:

1.Caloric Deficit: Weight loss is achieved when you consume fewer calories than your body burns. This is known as a caloric deficit. Nutrition plays a key role in creating this deficit by providing you with the right balance of macronutrients (carbohydrates, proteins, and fats) and micronutrients (vitamins, minerals, and antioxidants) while keeping calories in check.

2. Satiety and appetite control: Proper nutrition can help you feel satisfied and full for longer periods of time, reducing the chances of overeating or snacking on unhealthy foods. High-fiber foods, lean proteins, and healthy fats are all known to promote satiety and control appetite, helping you stick to your weight loss goals.

3. Metabolism boost: Certain foods and nutrients can boost your metabolism, helping your body burn calories more efficiently. For example, protein has a higher thermic effect of food, meaning it requires more energy to digest compared to carbohydrates or fats. Including protein in your meals can increase your metabolic rate and aid in weight loss.

4. **Blood sugar regulation:** Stable blood sugar levels are crucial for weight loss. When blood sugar spikes and crashes, it can lead to cravings, overeating, and fluctuations in energy levels. A well-balanced diet that includes complex carbohydrates, lean proteins, and healthy fats can help regulate blood sugar, keeping cravings at bay and providing steady energy levels throughout the day.

5. Muscle preservation: When you are in a calorie deficit, your body may start breaking down muscle tissue for energy. Proper nutrition, particularly adequate protein intake, can help preserve muscle mass and prevent muscle loss during weight loss. This is important as muscle contributes to an increased metabolism and overall strength.

6. Nutrient density: When aiming for weight loss, it is important to provide your body with all the necessary nutrients it needs to function optimally. Choosing nutrient-dense foods such as fruits, vegetables, whole grains, lean proteins, and healthy fats ensures that you are getting the right balance of vitamins, minerals, and antioxidants, even while in a calorie deficit.

7.Mindful eating and lifestyle change:
Weight loss is not a short-term fix but a long-term commitment to a healthier lifestyle. Nutrition teaches you to become more mindful of the foods you eat, their impact on your body, and how they make you feel. It helps in making better food choices, building healthy eating habits, and creating lasting lifestyle changes.

While nutrition is a powerful tool for weight loss, it is important to remember that every individual is unique and there is no one-size-fits-all approach to nutrition. Consulting with a registered dietitian or nutritionist can help you create a personalized and sustainable plan that meets your specific needs and goals.

the power of nutrition in weight loss cannot be overstated. By focusing on a well-balanced and nutrient-rich diet, you can achieve sustainable weight loss, improve your overall health, and establish a lifelong commitment to healthy eating habits.

Finding the Right Balance

Finding the right balance in weight loss is crucial for achieving long-term success and maintaining a healthy lifestyle. It involves a combination of various factors like proper nutrition, regular exercise, adequate rest, and managing stress levels. This comprehensive guide will help you understand the importance of balance in weight loss and provide practical tips to achieve it.

2. Balanced Nutrition:

Proper nutrition is vital for weight loss and overall health. While it's essential to create a calorie deficit to lose weight, it's equally important to fuel your body with balanced and nutritious food. Include a variety of fruits, vegetables, lean proteins, whole grains, and healthy fats in your diet. Avoid crash diets or extreme calorie restrictions, as they can negatively impact your metabolism and overall health. Opt for portion control, mindful eating, and balanced meal planning to achieve sustainable weight loss.

3. Regular Exercise:

Exercise plays a significant role in weight loss by burning calories, increasing metabolism, and improving cardiovascular health. Aim for a combination of cardiovascular exercises (walking, running, cycling) and strength training (weight lifting, resistance bands) to boost your weight loss journey. Be consistent with your exercise routine and gradually increase the intensity and duration to challenge your body. Additionally, incorporate activities you enjoy like dancing, swimming, or playing a sport to make it more enjoyable and sustainable.

4. Adequate Rest and Recovery:

Rest and recovery are often overlooked aspects of weight loss. Lack of sleep and chronic stress can sabotage your weight loss efforts by increasing cravings, imbalancing hormones, and slowing down metabolism. Aim for 7-8 hours of quality sleep every night and practice stress management techniques like meditation, yoga, deep breathing exercises, or engaging in hobbies to promote relaxation and well-being.

5. Mindful Eating:

Practicing mindful eating is essential for finding balance in weight loss. By paying attention to your body's hunger and fullness cues, you can avoid overeating and make healthier food choices. Eat slowly, savor each bite, and listen to your body's signals of fullness. Avoid distractions like TV, phone, or computer while eating, as it can lead to mindless eating.

6. Hydration:

Staying adequately hydrated is important for weight loss as it helps in boosting metabolism, reducing water retention, and controlling cravings. Drink at least 8 cups of water per day and opt for water instead of sugary drinks or sodas. You can also include green tea, herbal tea, or infused water for variety and additional health benefits.

7. Emotional and Mental Well-being:

Weight loss is not just about physical changes but also about emotional and mental well-being. Address emotional eating patterns, stress, and any underlying psychological factors that may be affecting your weight loss journey. Seek support from friends, family, or a professional counselor if needed. Practice self-care activities like journaling, meditation, or engaging in hobbies to reduce stress and promote emotional well-being.

8. Tracking Progress:

Keep track of your progress to stay motivated and make necessary adjustments. Monitor your weight, measurements, food intake, exercise routine, and emotions associated with your weight loss journey. Regularly reassess your goals and make modifications to your plan if required. Celebrate small achievements and achievements other than the number on the scale, like increased energy levels, improved confidence, or better sleep quality.

9. Long-term Sustainability:

Finding the right balance in weight loss is not just about achieving short-term goals but also about maintaining long-term sustainability. Avoid restrictive diets or quick fixes that are not sustainable in the long run. Instead, focus on making gradual lifestyle changes that you can maintain for a lifetime. Adopt healthy habits, create a supportive environment, and seek professional guidance if needed to ensure long-term success.

finding the right balance in weight loss is crucial for achieving sustainable results and maintaining a healthy lifestyle. It requires a combination of balanced nutrition, regular exercise, adequate rest, stress management, and addressing emotional and mental well-being. By following these tips, you can create a holistic approach to weight loss and improve your overall health and well-being. Remember, it's a journey, and finding the right balance may take time, patience, and self-compassion.

MINDFULNESS

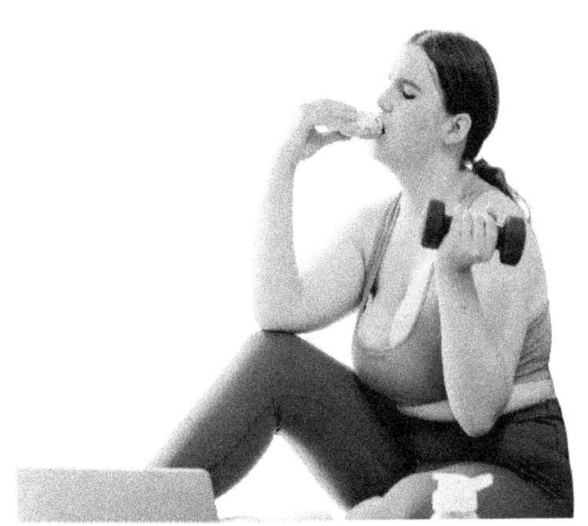

EATING

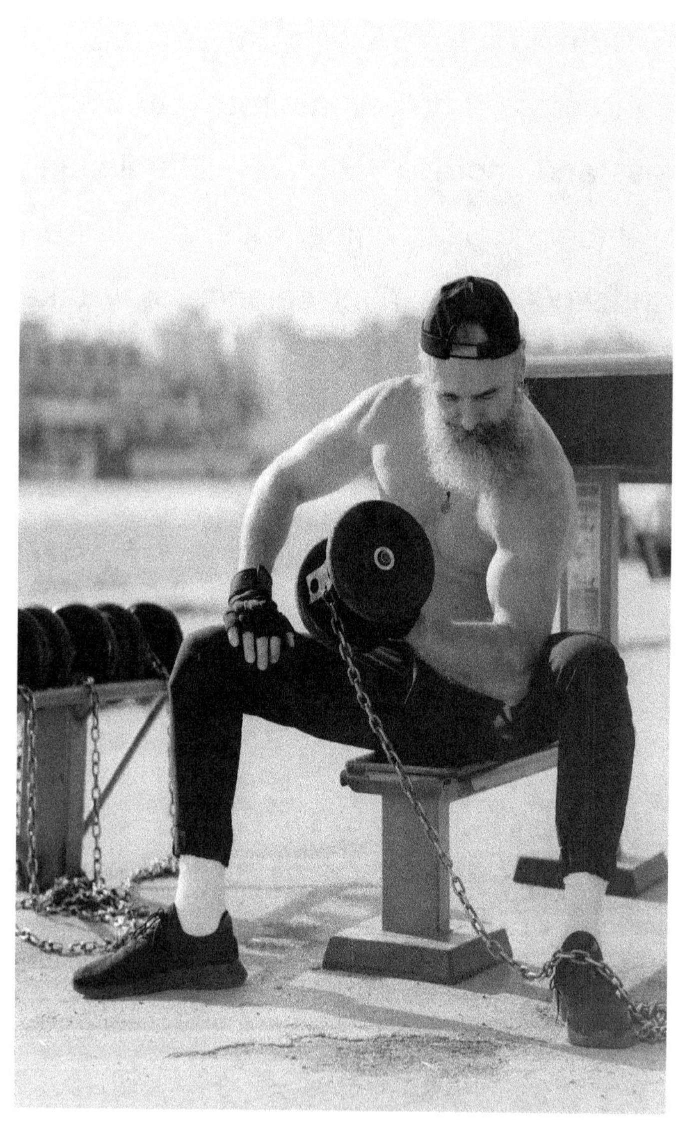

Chapter 7: The Transformation

Transformation is a powerful and life-changing journey, especially when it comes to weight loss. It involves not only shedding pounds but also developing a healthy lifestyle, finding self-confidence, and achieving long-term success. To embark on this journey, it is important to have a well-thought-out weight loss success guide that encompasses various aspects of physical, mental, and emotional well-being. In this comprehensive content, we will explore the different components of such a guide to help individuals achieve their weight loss goals and maintain a healthy lifestyle.

1. Set Clear and Realistic Goals: The first step towards any successful transformation is setting clear and achievable goals. It is essential to evaluate your current weight, body composition, and overall health to determine a realistic target. Setting small milestones along the way can help keep you motivated and focused on the bigger picture.

2. Educate Yourself: Understanding the science behind weight loss is crucial. Educate yourself on the principles of calorie intake, macronutrients, portion control, and the importance of regular physical activity. This knowledge will empower you to make informed decisions about food choices, exercise routines, and lifestyle changes.

3.Create a Healthy and Balanced Diet: A well-balanced diet plays a vital role in weight loss. Focus on consuming nutrient-dense foods that provide essential vitamins, minerals, and fiber. Incorporate a variety of fruits, vegetables, lean proteins, whole grains, and healthy fats into your diet. Avoid processed foods, sugary snacks, and excessive intake of refined carbohydrates.

4. Practice Portion Control: Portion control is key to managing calorie intake. Be mindful of your portion sizes and use tools like measuring cups or a food scale to ensure accurate measurements. Consider serving meals on smaller plates, which can help create an illusion of a larger portion. Avoid eating directly from the package, as it can lead to mindless overeating.

5. Hydration: Staying hydrated is essential for overall health and weight loss. Drinking an adequate amount of water not only helps maintain proper bodily functions but can also curb hunger and reduce calorie intake. Aim to drink at least eight glasses of water per day and replace sugary drinks with healthier alternatives like herbal teas or infused water.

6. Regular Physical Activity: Incorporating regular exercise into your routine is crucial for weight loss success. Find activities you enjoy, such as jogging, swimming, cycling, or attending fitness classes. Aim for a combination of cardiovascular exercises, strength training, and flexibility workouts. Start with manageable timeframes and gradually increase the intensity and duration to avoid injuries and burnout.

7. Monitor Progress: Keep track of your progress by regularly weighing yourself, taking measurements, and keeping a food and exercise journal. This self-monitoring allows you to identify patterns, evaluate your progress, and make necessary adjustments to your routine. Celebrate small victories along the way to stay motivated.

8. Seek Support: Surround yourself with a strong support system that understands and encourages your weight loss journey. Join support groups, online communities, or find an accountability partner who can provide guidance, motivation, and share experiences.

9. Prioritize Sleep: Quality sleep is often overlooked but crucial for weight loss success. Lack of sleep can lead to imbalances in hunger hormones and increased cravings for unhealthy foods. Aim for 7-9 hours of quality sleep every night to support your weight loss efforts.

10. Manage Stress: Stress can hinder weight loss progress by increasing cortisol levels, which promotes fat storage. Incorporate stress management techniques like meditation, deep breathing exercises, yoga, or engaging in hobbies to reduce stress levels and prevent emotional eating.

11. Practice Mindful Eating: Mindful eating involves paying attention to the present moment while eating, being aware of physical hunger, and recognizing fullness cues. Slow down, savor your food, chew thoroughly, and listen to your body's signals. This practice can help prevent overeating and foster a healthy relationship with food.

12. Embrace Consistency and Patience: Weight loss is not an overnight process; it requires consistency, dedication, and patience. Embrace the journey, focus on creating sustainable habits, and remember that the results will come with time if you stay committed.

13. Celebrate Non-scale Victories: While the number on the scale is an indicator of progress, it shouldn't be your only measure of success. Celebrate non-scale victories such as increased energy levels, improved flexibility, fitting into smaller clothing sizes, or achieving fitness milestones.

14. Avoid Fad Diets and Quick Fixes: Be cautious of quick-fix diets promising rapid weight loss. They often lead to unsustainable results, nutrient deficiencies, and can even have long-term negative effects on your metabolism. Instead, focus on creating a well-rounded, healthy eating plan that you can maintain for a lifetime.

15. Maintain Consistency Beyond Weight Loss: The ultimate goal of any weight loss success guide is to maintain a healthy lifestyle beyond the initial transformation. Once you reach your target weight, shift your focus towards weight maintenance, regular physical activity, and continued self-care.

embarking on a weight loss transformation requires a comprehensive and well-thought-out plan. By setting realistic goals, educating yourself, creating a balanced diet, incorporating regular exercise, seeking support, and implementing stress management techniques, you can achieve long-term weight loss success. Remember to celebrate your progress, embrace consistency, and prioritize overall well-being to maintain a healthy lifestyle beyond the transformation journey.

Incorporating Exercise for a Healthy Lifestyle

Incorporating exercise into a healthy lifestyle is an essential aspect of any weight loss journey. Exercise not only burns calories, but it also helps to build and tone muscles, increase metabolism, improve cardiovascular health, and boost overall mood and well-being.

There are several key factors to consider when incorporating exercise into a weight loss plan:

1. Choose activities you enjoy: Finding physical activities that are enjoyable and fun will increase the likelihood of long-term adherence. This may include activities such as walking, jogging, biking, swimming, dancing, or participating in group fitness classes.

3. Create a balanced routine: A well-rounded exercise routine should include a combination of cardiovascular exercise, strength training, and flexibility exercises. Cardiovascular exercise helps to burn calories and improve heart health, strength training builds muscle and boosts metabolism, and flexibility exercises increase range of motion and prevent injuries.

3. Start slow and gradually increase intensity: It is important to start with low to moderate intensity exercises and gradually increase the intensity and duration over time. This allows the body to adapt and reduces the risk of injury. It is also important to listen to one's body and take rest days when needed.

4. Incorporate variety: Adding variety to an exercise routine not only prevents boredom but also challenges different muscles and prevents plateaus. Trying new activities, incorporating different forms of cardio and strength training, and participating in group fitness classes can help to keep the routine fresh and exciting.

5. Make exercise a daily habit: Consistency is key when it comes to exercise. Aim to make exercise a daily habit by scheduling it into the daily routine and prioritizing it. Finding a time of day that works best, whether it is in the morning, during lunch breaks, or in the evening, can help to make exercise a consistent part of the routine.

6. Seek professional guidance: If new to exercise or unsure of where to start, seeking guidance from a certified personal trainer or fitness professional can be beneficial. They can provide personalized exercise programs, ensure proper form and technique, and provide motivation and accountability.

7. Combine exercise with a balanced diet: While exercise is an important component of weight loss, it is essential to also focus on nutrition and a balanced diet. Pairing exercise with a diet rich in whole foods, lean proteins, fruits, vegetables, and healthy fats will maximize weight loss efforts.

8.Stay motivated:

Maintaining motivation is crucial for long-term success. Set short-term and long-term goals, track progress, reward achievements, find a workout buddy or support group, and switch up the routine to stay motivated and committed.

9.Listen to the body: It is important to listen to one's body and make adjustments as needed. If feeling fatigued or experiencing pain, it may be necessary to take a rest day or modify the exercise routine. Rest and recovery are just as important for performance and overall health as exercise itself.

Incorporating exercise into a healthy lifestyle is a key component of weight loss. By setting realistic goals, choosing enjoyable activities, creating a balanced routine, starting slow and gradually increasing intensity, incorporating variety, making exercise a daily habit, seeking professional guidance, combining exercise with a balanced diet, staying motivated, and listening to the body, one can achieve sustainable weight loss and improve overall health and well-being.

Chapter 8: Mindset Matters

When it comes to achieving weight loss success, many people focus on the physical aspect of the journey – what to eat, how to exercise, and which strategies can help shed those extra pounds. While these factors are undoubtedly significant, one crucial element that often gets overlooked is the mindset. The way you think, feel, and approach weight loss plays a vital role in determining your success. In fact, having a positive mindset can be the driving force behind long-term, sustainable weight loss. In this guide, we will explore why mindset matters and provide strategies to develop a positive mindset for weight loss success.

Understanding the Mindset-Weight Loss Connection

1. Recognizing Your Current Mindset:
Before embarking on any weight loss journey, it is essential to evaluate your current mindset. Are you plagued by negative thoughts, self-doubt, or fear of failure? Or do you possess a growth mindset, believing in your ability to make positive changes? Self-reflection will help you identify any limiting beliefs or thought patterns that may hinder your progress and allow you to take the necessary steps to change them.

2. The Power of Positive Thinking:
Positive thinking is not just an airy concept; it has a significant impact on our actions and outcomes. When you believe in yourself and your ability to achieve your weight loss goals, you are more likely to take consistent, positive actions. On the other hand, if you constantly focus on your failures, setbacks, or negative aspects of your body, it can become a self-fulfilling prophecy that hinders your progress. Embracing positive thinking and

cultivating a growth mindset will be a game-changer on your weight loss journey.

3. Overcoming Self-Sabotage:

One of the biggest obstacles to weight loss success is self-sabotage. This typically occurs when our actions contradict our desires or when we engage in negative behaviors that hinder progress. Recognizing the underlying reasons behind self-sabotaging behavior, such as emotional eating or lack of self-discipline, is crucial. By developing self-awareness and adopting positive coping strategies, such as mindful eating or stress reduction techniques, you can overcome self-sabotage and stay on track towards your weight loss goals.

Developing a Positive Mindset for Weight Loss Success

1. Set Realistic Goals:
While it is essential to aim high and challenge yourself, setting unrealistic goals can set you up for failure and disappointment. Instead, set realistic and achievable goals that align with your lifestyle, capabilities, and timeframe. Celebrate small victories along the way, and don't underestimate the power of progress, no matter how small.

2. Practice Self-Compassion:
Weight loss journeys can be challenging, and setbacks are bound to happen. Rather than beating yourself up or engaging in negative self-talk, practice self-compassion. Treat yourself with kindness, understanding, and forgiveness. Remember that no one is perfect, and learning from setbacks is an essential part of growth.

3. Surround Yourself with Positivity:

The company we keep greatly influences our mindset. Surround yourself with supportive individuals who share your goals or have already achieved weight loss success. Engage in communities or support groups that provide encouragement and inspiration. Additionally, expose yourself to positive affirmations, motivational books, podcasts, or educational resources that reinforce a positive mindset.

4. Focus on Non-Scale Victories:

While weight loss is often measured by numbers on a scale, it is crucial to acknowledge non-scale victories. Pay attention to how your body feels, how your clothes fit, or your improved energy levels. Celebrate these accomplishments, as they are an indication of progress and success, regardless of what the scale says.

5.Practice Mindfulness and Emotional Awareness:

Developing mindfulness and emotional awareness can significantly impact your relationship with food and your body. Be present and fully engage in your meals, savoring each bite and listening to your body's hunger and fullness cues. When confronted with emotional eating triggers, practice self-awareness, and find alternative coping strategies like exercise, journaling, or talking to a supportive friend.

In the quest for weight loss success, mindset matters. Cultivating a positive mindset, embracing self-compassion, setting realistic goals, and practicing mindfulness are all essential components. By acknowledging the power of your thoughts and beliefs, you can create a foundation for lasting change and achieve your weight loss goals with confidence and long-term success. Remember, your mindset is the key to unlock your fullest potential.

Shifting Perspectives and Cultivating Self-Love

When embarking on a weight loss journey, it's common to solely focus on the physical aspects of shedding pounds. While physical exercise and proper nutrition are crucial components, it's equally important to shift our perspectives and cultivate self-love along the way. Shifting perspectives involves changing our mindset, attitudes, and beliefs about ourselves, our bodies, and our overall well-being. Cultivating self-love is about fostering a deep sense of acceptance, compassion, and kindness towards ourselves. These two elements are not only important for successful weight loss but also for maintaining a healthy and balanced life in the long run.

Shifting perspectives plays a vital role in transforming our relationship with food and exercise. Instead of viewing weight loss as a punishment or a means to an end, we can adopt a more positive and empowering perspective. We can shift our focus to the numerous benefits of losing weight, such as increased energy levels, improved physical health, enhanced self-confidence, and a greater sense of well-being. Instead of viewing exercise as a chore, we can start seeing it as an opportunity to move our bodies, relieve stress, and improve our overall mental state. By shifting our perspectives, we can develop a more positive and sustainable approach to weight loss, making it a lifelong journey rather than a short-term goal.

Cultivating self-love is perhaps one of the most crucial aspects of a weight loss journey. Low self-esteem and negative self-talk often contribute to unhealthy habits and a cycle of emotional eating. When we cultivate self-love, we develop a stronger sense of self-worth, which drives us to make healthier choices. Instead of using food as a coping mechanism, we learn to nourish our bodies with wholesome and nutritious options. By practicing self-love, we also become more attuned to our body's needs, recognizing when we are truly hungry versus eating out of boredom or emotional distress. Through self-love, we can break free from the cycle of guilt and shame often associated with weight loss and truly embrace a halthier lifestyle.

Shifting perspectives and cultivating self-love are not overnight transformations. They require consistent practice and dedication. Here are some strategies to incorporate into your weight loss journey:

1. Challenge negative thoughts and beliefs: Notice when negative thoughts or beliefs arise about yourself or your body. Replace these thoughts with positive affirmations and remind yourself of your worth and potential.

2. Practice self-compassion: Treat yourself with kindness and understanding, especially during setbacks or difficult moments. Remember that you are human, and progress takes time.

3. Surround yourself with a positive support system: Seek out friends, family, or a weight loss community that uplifts and encourages you. Avoid toxic relationships or environments that undermine your self-love and progress.

4. Focus on non-scale victories: Instead of solely relying on the number on the scale, celebrate other achievements such as increased energy levels, improved sleep, or feeling stronger during workouts.

5. Incorporate self-care activities into your routine: Engage in activities that bring you joy and help you relax, such as taking baths, practicing yoga, reading, or spending time in nature. Taking care of your mental and emotional well-being is just as important as physical exercise.

6. Set realistic and attainable goals: Break down your weight loss journey into smaller, achievable goals. Celebrate each milestone along the way, reinforcing your self-love and motivation.

Shifting perspectives and cultivating self-love are essential for a successful weight loss journey. By changing our mindset, embracing self-acceptance, and practicing self-compassion, we can transform not only our bodies but also our overall well-being. Remember, weight loss is not just about the numbers; it's about nurturing a healthy mind, body, and soul.

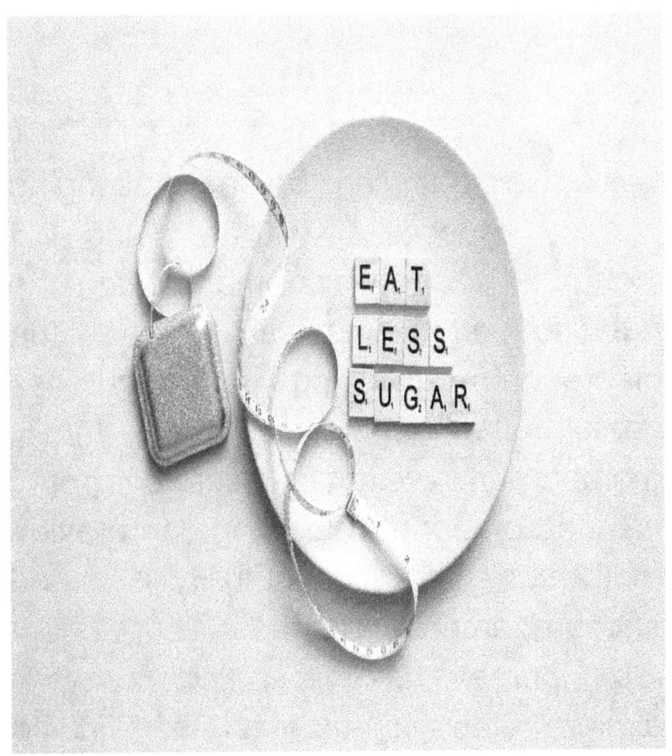

Chapter 9: Finding Support

Losing weight can be a challenging journey, especially if you are going at it alone. It is often said that having the right support system can make all the difference in achieving your weight loss goals. Whether it is a friend, family member, or a weight loss support group, having someone to lean on can provide motivation, accountability, and encouragement throughout your weight loss journey. In this article, we will explore the importance of finding support in a weight loss guide and provide tips on how to find the right support system for you.

1. Motivation and Accountability:

Having someone to share your weight loss goals with can provide the motivation and accountability needed to stay on track. When you have someone cheering you on and holding you accountable for your actions, it becomes easier to stay focused and committed to your weight loss plan. Furthermore, having someone who shares a similar goal can provide the motivation you need to push through when times get tough.

2. Expert Guidance:

A weight loss guide or support group can provide you with expert guidance and advice that can help you navigate through your weight loss journey effectively. These guides often have experienced professionals who can provide you with personalized meal plans, exercise routines, and tips on how to overcome common hurdles that may arise during weight loss. By having access to this knowledge and expertise, you can make informed decisions and avoid common pitfalls that often hinder progress.

3. Emotional Support:

Weight loss is not just physical; it is also an emotional journey. There may be times when you feel discouraged, frustrated, or overwhelmed. Having someone who understands your struggles, listens to your concerns, and offers emotional support can make a world of difference. A supportive friend, family member, or support group can be a safe space for you to vent, share your feelings, and seek validation. This emotional support can help you stay motivated and mentally strong throughout your weight loss journey.

4. Practical Tips and Advice:

In addition to emotional support, a weight loss support system can provide you with practical tips and advice. These tips may include healthy recipes, meal planning techniques, exercise routines, and lifestyle modifications. By having access to a variety of tips and advice, you can find what works best for you and implement them into your daily routine.

5. Celebration of Successes:

When you reach a milestone or achieve a weight loss goal, having someone to celebrate your success with can be incredibly rewarding. Sharing your achievements with others who understand the hard work and dedication it takes to lose weight can be a great source of motivation and encouragement. Additionally, celebrating your successes can reinforce positive behaviors and help you stay motivated to continue your weight loss journey.

Tips for Finding the Right Support System:

1. Identify Your Needs: Before seeking support, take the time to reflect on what you need the most. Are you looking for an accountability partner? Do you need emotional support? Are you seeking expert guidance? Understanding your needs will help you find the right support system that can meet those requirements.

2. Seek Support from Friends and Family: Start by reaching out to friends and family members who you trust and feel comfortable sharing your weight loss journey with. They may be willing to join you on your journey or provide the support you need.

3. Join a Weight Loss Support Group: Many communities and online platforms offer weight loss support groups where individuals with similar goals come together to share experiences, seek advice, and provide each other with support. Look for a group that aligns with your needs and values and consider joining them.

4. Work with a Personal Trainer or Nutritionist: If you prefer a more personalized approach, consider working with a personal trainer or nutritionist who can guide you through your weight loss journey. They can provide expert advice, set realistic goals, and hold you accountable for your actions.

5. Utilize Online Resources: There are many online platforms, forums, and blogs dedicated to weight loss and healthy living. These platforms can provide a wealth of information, support, and inspiration. Consider joining a weight loss forum or following blogs that resonate with you.

 finding support in a weight loss guide is crucial for success. Having a support system can provide motivation, accountability, emotional support, expert guidance, practical tips, and a space to celebrate your successes. By seeking out the right support system for you, you can greatly increase your chances of achieving your weight loss goals and maintaining a healthy lifestyle.

Building a Network of Accountability

Are you tired of starting a weight loss regimen only to give up after a few weeks? Do you struggle with staying accountable to your goals and maintaining the motivation to achieve them? If so, joining a network of accountability on a weight loss guide might be the solution you've been looking for.

Accountability is a powerful tool when it comes to achieving any goal, and weight loss is no exception. When you have a network of like-minded individuals who are also on a weight loss journey, it becomes easier to stay committed and motivated. They are there to support and encourage you every step of the way, making the whole process much more enjoyable.

One of the key benefits of joining a network of accountability is that you have access to a group of people who understand your struggles and challenges. Losing weight can be difficult, and sometimes it feels like no one else truly understands what you're going through. However, being part of a network allows you to connect with others who are facing similar challenges and can relate to your journey.

In addition to emotional support, a network of accountability can provide practical guidance and resources. Many weight loss programs offer weekly or monthly check-ins where you can discuss your progress, challenges, and goals. These check-ins can help keep you on track and provide valuable insights and advice from experts or more experienced members of the network.

Furthermore, participating in a network of accountability allows you to set specific goals and milestones for yourself. When you publicly commit to your goals, you feel a stronger sense of responsibility to follow through. It's no longer just about letting yourself down; it's about letting the entire network down. This added pressure can be the extra push you need to stay motivated and focused.

Another advantage of an accountability network is that it provides opportunities for friendly competition and healthy challenges. Many programs organize challenges or contests within the group, such as a step challenge, weight loss challenge, or healthy recipe challenge. These friendly competitions can not only make weight loss more fun but also boost your motivation to perform better and achieve your goals.

Finally, being part of a network of accountability is a great way to celebrate your successes and achievements. When you hit a milestone or reach a goal, you can share your excitement with the group, and they will be there to celebrate with you. Having a supportive community to share your wins with can amplify the joy and sense of accomplishment, making the entire weight loss journey more rewarding.

 joining a network of accountability on a weight loss guide can be a game-changer for anyone struggling to stay motivated and achieve their weight loss goals. With emotional support, practical guidance, goal-setting opportunities, friendly competition, and celebration of successes, an accountability network provides the necessary tools to make your weight loss journey a success. So why go at it alone? Find a network of accountability and start achieving your weight loss goals today.

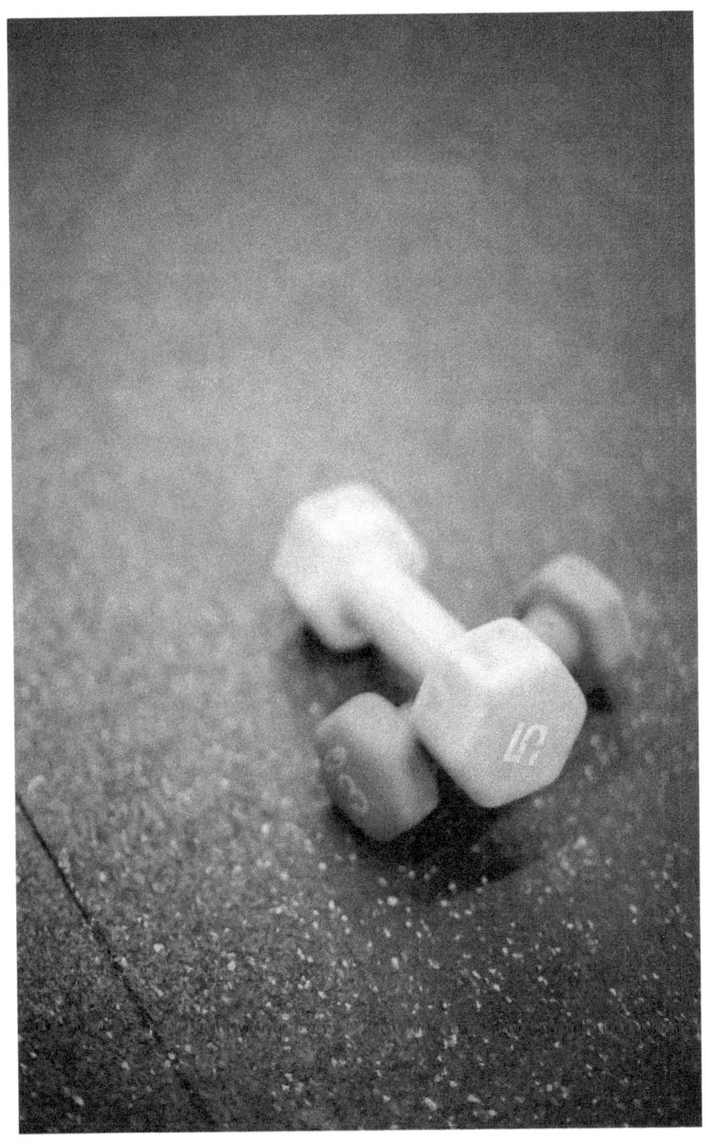

Chapter 10

Maintaining the Momentum Strategies for Long-Term Success

Losing weight is a tremendous achievement, but maintaining the momentum and staying on track for the long-term is equally important. Here are some strategies that can help you maintain your weight loss success and achieve long-term sustainable results.

1. Stick to Healthy Eating Habits: It's important to continue making healthy food choices even after achieving your weight loss goals. Maintain a balanced diet by incorporating plenty of fruits, vegetables, lean proteins, and whole grains into your meals. Avoid or limit processed foods, sugary snacks, and excessive junk food consumption. Remember to practice portion control to prevent overeating.

2. Stay Active: Exercise plays a vital role in maintaining weight loss. Aim for at least 150 minutes of moderate-intensity aerobic activity per week, or 75 minutes of vigorous-intensity aerobic activity. Find physical activities that you enjoy and make them a regular part of your routine. Incorporate strength training exercises to build muscle, which can help increase your metabolism and burn more calories.

3. Track Your Progress: Regularly monitoring your weight and documenting your progress can help you stay accountable. Keep a food journal or use a tracking app to record your daily food intake. This will help you identify any patterns or triggers that might lead to overeating. Continuously tracking your progress can help you identify areas where you might need to make adjustments and stay motivated.

4. Seek Support: Surrounding yourself with a Support system can make a significant difference in maintaining weight loss. Join a weight loss support group, enroll in a local fitness class, or seek the help of a registered dietitian or weight loss coach. Having someone to share your journey with, exchange tips, and hold you accountable can greatly enhance your chances of maintaining long-term success.

5. Celebrate Non-Scale Victories: Remember that success is not solely measured by the numbers on the scale. Celebrate the non-scale victories, such as having more energy, fitting into smaller clothes, or noticing improved mental clarity. These victories can be just as rewarding and motivating as losing weight.

By following these strategies, you can maintain the momentum and achieve long-term success on your weight loss journey. Remember, it's a lifestyle change, not a quick fix. Stay consistent, be patient with yourself, and embrace the journey to a healthier, happier you.

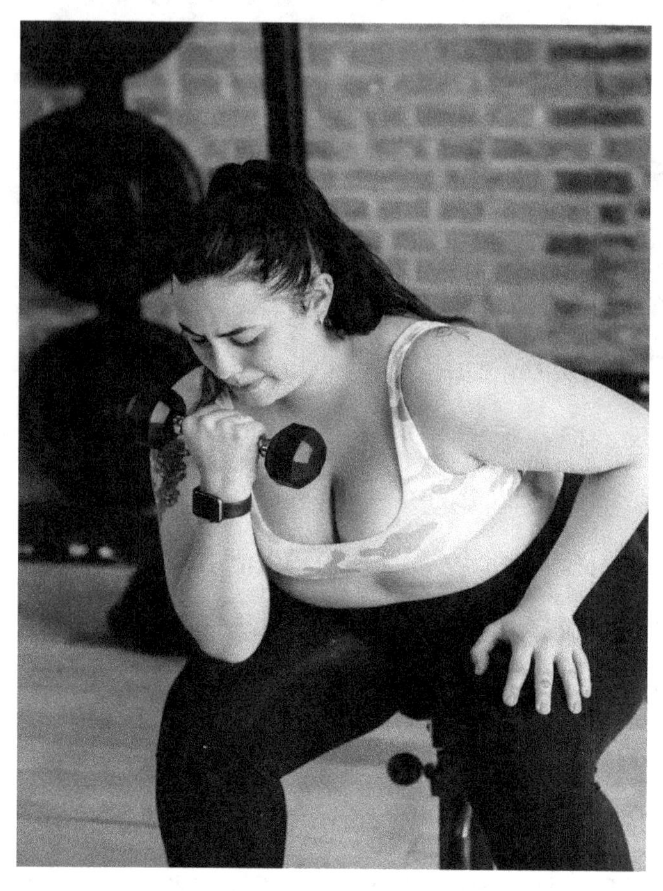

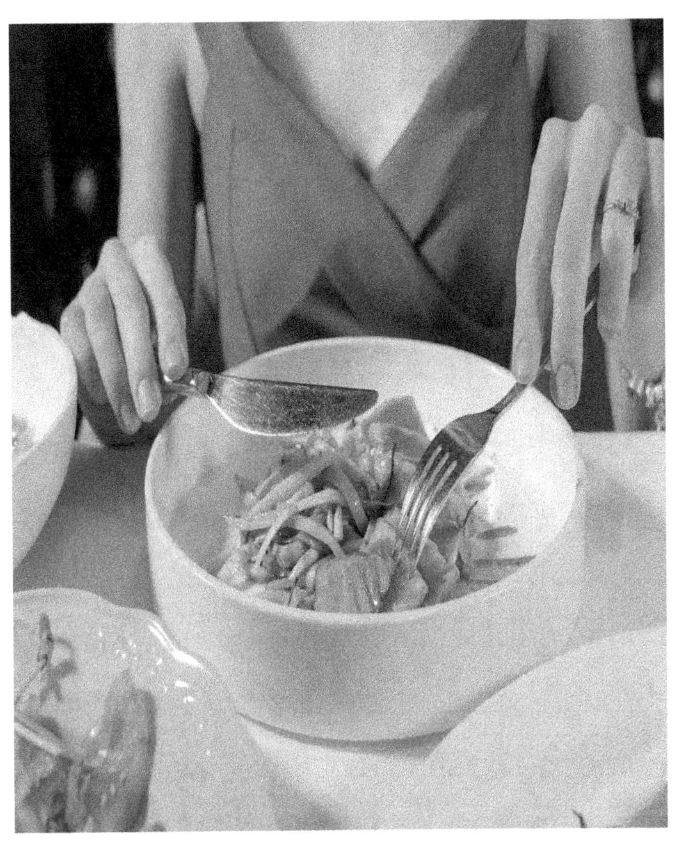

STICK HEALTHY

EATING HABITS

Chapter 11

Celebrating Milestones Appreciating the Journey and the Wins

Losing weight is no easy feat. It requires dedication, willpower, and commitment. It involves making healthier choices, changing lifestyle habits, and pushing through obstacles. That's why when someone achieves their weight loss goals, it's important to celebrate the milestones and appreciate the journey that led them there.

This book Weight loss success stories are a testament to the incredible transformations that individuals can achieve. These stories not only inspire others who are on their own weight loss journey, but they also serve as a reminder of the hard work and perseverance that goes into accomplishing such a feat. Whether someone has lost 10 pounds or 100 pounds, each milestone should be acknowledged and celebrated.

Celebrating milestones along the weight loss journey serves several purposes.

Firstly, it helps to boost motivation and confidence. Recognizing progress and the positive changes that have taken place can provide the much-needed encouragement to keep going. It's a chance for individuals to reflect on how far they've come and remind themselves that they are capable of achieving their goals. Appreciating the journey that led to weight loss success is just as important as celebrating the milestones. It's about recognizing the effort, determination, and self-discipline that was exerted. Whether it was sticking to a healthy meal plan, hitting the gym consistently, or overcoming emotional obstacles, each step along the journey contributes to the overall success. Acknowledging this journey can help individuals develop a sense of pride and accomplishment, enhancing their overall well-being.

Furthermore, celebrating and appreciating weight loss milestones can inspire and motivate others who are also on a quest to lose weight. By sharing success stories, individuals can offer support, advice, and encouragement to others who may be facing similar challenges. This creates a sense of community and camaraderie among individuals with similar goals.

celebrating milestones and appreciating the journey on weight loss success stories is essential. It provides motivation, boosts confidence, and encourages others who are on their own journey. It's a chance to reflect on progress and remind oneself of the incredible transformation that has taken place..

Chapter 12: Beyond the Scale

Weight loss is a journey that is often filled with challenges, setbacks, and doubts. However, there are countless success stories out there that prove that it is possible to overcome these obstacles and achieve remarkable transformations. These stories not only provide motivation for those on a weight loss journey but also serve as a reminder that weight loss is not just about the numbers on a scale but about overall well-being and self-improvement.

Beyond the Scale is a program by Weight Watchers that focuses on a holistic approach to weight loss. It goes beyond the traditional focus on weight and emphasizes the importance of fostering a healthy relationship with food, promoting physical activity, and prioritizing mental well-being. This approach has resulted in countless success stories of individuals who have achieved significant weight loss and transformed their lives for the better.

One such success story is that of Amber, who struggled with weight her entire life and had tried numerous diets and weight loss programs with little success. When she joined Weight Watchers and adopted the Beyond the Scale approach, she found the support and tools she needed to make sustainable changes to her lifestyle. Within a year, Amber lost over 80 pounds and gained a newfound confidence and appreciation for her body. She attributes her success not only to the program's focus on healthy eating and exercise but also to the emphasis on self-acceptance and positive mindset.

Another inspiring story is that of Mark, who had battled with obesity for most of his adult life. With a combination of poor eating habits and a sedentary lifestyle, Mark's weight had spiraled out of control, leading to various health issues and a negative impact on his mental well-being. Joining Weight Watchers and embracing the Beyond the Scale philosophy was a turning point for Mark. He learned to make healthier choices, started incorporating exercise into his daily routine, and sought therapy to address the emotional aspects of his weight struggles. Over time, Mark lost over 150 pounds and regained his health, happiness, and confidence.

Beyond the Scale is not just about weight loss, but also about overall health and well-being. It encourages individuals to focus on non-scale victories, such as increased energy levels, improved sleep, reduced stress, and enhanced self-esteem. These achievements are just as important as the numbers on a scale and help create a positive mindset for long-term success.

One of the key components of Beyond the Scale is the SmartPoints system, which assigns a value to every food and beverage based on its nutritional content. This system encourages members to make healthier choices by prioritizing foods that are lower in sugar, saturated fat, and calories while being higher in protein and fiber. This approach enables individuals to still enjoy their favorite foods while fostering a balanced and nutritious diet.

Additionally, Beyond the Scale emphasizes the importance of regular physical activity. It encourages members to find activities they enjoy and make them a part of their daily routine. Whether it's going for a walk, taking a dance class, or lifting weights, incorporating exercise into one's lifestyle not only aids in weight loss but also improves cardiovascular health, strengthens muscles, and enhances overall well-being.

The support and community aspect of Beyond the Scale cannot be understated. Weight Watchers provides members with access to a network of like-minded individuals who are on their own weight loss journey. Whether it's attending weekly meetings, participating in online forums, or connecting through social media, the support and accountability from others can be a powerful motivator in achieving weight loss success.

Beyond the Scale is a program by Weight Watchers that focuses on a holistic approach to weight loss, emphasizing healthy eating, regular physical activity, and positive mindset.

The success stories of individuals who have embraced this approach serve as an inspiration for others on their weight loss journey. These stories highlight that weight loss is not just about the numbers on a scale, but about overall well-being, self-improvement, and a sustainable lifestyle change. Through the support of the Beyond the Scale community and the adoption of a healthier mindset, individuals can achieve remarkable transformations and live their best lives.

Embracing a Healthy and Balanced Life

Weight loss success stories are often seen as the ultimate goal for individuals seeking to embrace a healthy and balanced life. These stories inspire and motivate others, showing them that with dedication, determination, and the right mindset, they too can achieve their weight loss goals and live a healthier life.

Embracing a healthy and balanced life goes beyond just losing weight. It means adopting a mindset that focuses on nourishing the body, exercising regularly, and finding a balance between work, family, and self-care. It is about making sustainable lifestyle changes that promote overall well-being and happiness.

One of the keys to achieving a healthy and balanced life is understanding that weight loss is not a one-size-fits-all approach. What works for one person may not work for another. Therefore, it is important to find a weight loss plan or strategy that aligns with individual goals, preferences, and lifestyle.

There are countless weight loss success stories out there, each unique in its own way. Some individuals may have lost weight through strict dieting and intense exercise routines, while others may have found success through mindful eating, adopting a plant-based diet, or incorporating more movement into their daily lives.

Regardless of the path taken, weight loss success stories often involve a combination of healthy eating, regular physical activity, and a positive and determined mindset. It is important to establish realistic goals and expectations and to celebrate each milestone along the way.

Embracing a healthy and balanced life also involves taking care of oneself on a mental and emotional level. This includes managing stress, getting enough sleep, practicing self-care activities, and surrounding oneself with a supportive and positive environment.

Additionally, it is important to cultivate an attitude of self-love and acceptance throughout the weight loss journey. Striving for progress, not perfection, and recognizing that setbacks and plateaus are a natural part of the process can help individuals stay motivated and focused on their goals.

It is also valuable to seek support and guidance from professionals or support groups. Nutritionists, personal trainers, therapists or counselors, and weight loss support groups can provide expert advice, accountability, and encouragement along the journey. Having a strong support system can make a significant difference in staying committed to a healthy and balanced lifestyle.

embracing a healthy and balanced life is a lifelong journey that involves taking care of the physical, mental, and emotional aspects of oneself. Weight loss can be a part of this journey, but it is important to remember that true success comes from creating sustainable habits and prioritizing one's overall well-being. By adopting a positive mindset, setting realistic goals, and seeking support and guidance when needed, anyone can achieve their weight loss and overall health goals and live a fulfilling, healthy, and balanced life.

Conclusion

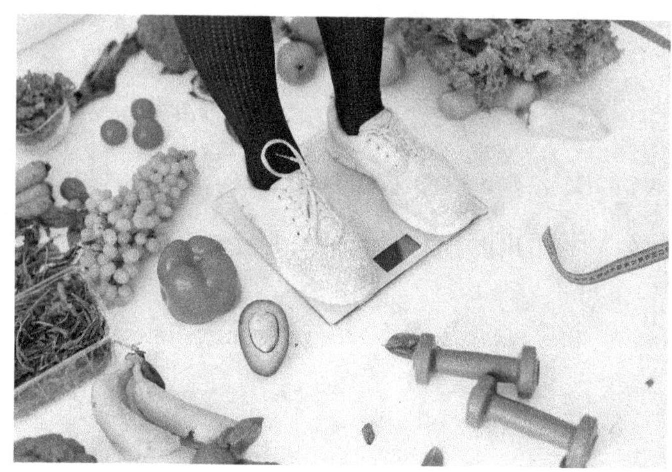

Choosing Health, Happiness, and a New Beginning

weight loss success stories featured in "Choosing Health, Happiness, and a New Beginning" provide inspiring and valuable insights into the journey of losing weight and transforming one's life. These stories demonstrate that with determination, dedication, and a positive mindset, anyone can achieve their weight loss goals and improve their overall health and happiness.

The individuals featured in these success stories have overcome various challenges, including emotional eating, lack of motivation, and a sedentary lifestyle. Through their perseverance and commitment to change, they have not only shed excess pounds but have also experienced an improved sense of self-esteem, increased energy levels, and a renewed zest for life.

One common theme that emerges from these stories is the importance of setting realistic goals and making sustainable lifestyle changes. Many of the participants emphasize the significance of making small, gradual changes to their diet and exercise routines, rather than resorting to extreme measures or fad diets. This approach ensures that the weight loss is not only effective but also sustainable in the long run.

Furthermore, these success stories highlight the crucial role of support systems in achieving weight loss goals. Many of the individuals attribute their success to the encouragement and guidance they received from friends, family, or professional trainers. This reinforces the notion that having a strong support network can make a significant difference in maintaining motivation and accountability.

Importantly, these narratives remind us that weight loss is not just about physical appearance but also about overall well-being. Participants frequently mention the positive impact of their weight loss on their mental and emotional health, as well as their relationships. They describe feeling more confident, happier, and more in control of their lives.

Overall, the weight loss success stories in "Choosing Health, Happiness, and a New Beginning" serve as powerful examples of how making conscious choices towards health and happiness can lead to transformative outcomes. Whether it is losing a significant amount of weight or simply adopting healthier habits, these narratives inspire us to believe in our own ability to change and choose a better life.

 As you read And seen inside this book I talked about setting a realistic goals of your self in many chapters,so Did want to see what means by that by Example?,if you want don't worry I have one book of my colleagues that definitely shows that for you in a pages less than 50, the book talk about how an American Rookie Qb star lead his team to victory without knowing All his teammates names, here's the Name of the book
Rookie QB Magic search it on Amazon board.

www.ingramcontent.com/pod-product-compliance
Lightning Source LLC
Chambersburg PA
CBHW050818260726
48660CB00004B/1500